Acting Edition

The Old Man and the Pool

by Mike Birbiglia

SAMUEL FRENCH

No one shall make any changes in this title(s) for the purpose of production. No part of this book may be reproduced, stored in a retrieval system, scanned, uploaded, or transmitted in any form, by any means, now known or yet to be invented, including mechanical, electronic, digital, photocopying, recording, videotaping, or otherwise, without the prior written permission of the publisher. No one shall share this title(s), or any part of this title(s), through any social media or file hosting websites.

For all inquiries regarding motion picture, television, online/digital and other media rights, please contact Concord Theatricals Corp.

MUSIC AND THIRD-PARTY MATERIALS USE NOTE

Licensees are solely responsible for obtaining formal written permission from copyright owners to use copyrighted music and/or other copyrighted third-party materials (e.g. artworks, logos) in the performance of this play and are strongly cautioned to do so. If no such permission is obtained by the licensee, then the licensee must use only original music and materials that the licensee owns and controls. Licensees are solely responsible and liable for clearances of all third-party copyrighted materials, including without limitation music, and shall indemnify the copyright owners of the play(s) and their licensing agent, Concord Theatricals Corp., against any costs, expenses, losses and liabilities arising from the use of such copyrighted third-party materials by licensees. For music, please contact the appropriate music licensing authority in your territory for the rights to any incidental music.

IMPORTANT BILLING AND CREDIT REQUIREMENTS

If you have obtained performance rights to this title, please refer to your licensing agreement for important billing and credit requirements.

THE OLD MAN AND THE POOL was originally produced by Center Theatre Group, and received its world premiere at the Mark Taper Forum in Los Angeles, CA, in 2022. It was written and performed by Mike Birbiglia. The production was directed by Seth Barrish, with scenic design by Beowulf Boritt, costumes design by Toni-Leslie James, lighting design by Aaron Copp, projection design by Hana S. Kim, and sound design by Kai Harada.

THE OLD MAN AND THE POOL was produced on Broadway by Sue Wagner, John Johnson, Patrick Catullo, Seaview, and Center Theatre Group and premiered at the Vivian Beaumont Theater on November 13, 2022. The cast and creative team were the same. The production stage manager was Laurie Goldfeder.

THE OLD MAN AND THE POOL was developed, in part, by Berkeley Repertory Theatre (Johanna Pfaelzer, Artistic Director; Tom Parrish, Managing Director) in 2021 and Steppenwolf Theatre Company (Glenn Davis and Audrey Francis, Artistic Directors; Brooke Flanagan, Executive Director) in 2022.

CHARACTER

MIKE

AUTHOR'S NOTE

I've written six solo plays over the last twenty years. *Sleepwalk With Me, My Girlfriend's Boyfriend, Thank God For Jokes, The New One, The Old Man and the Pool,* and *The Good Life.* These shows were all directed by Seth Barrish and staged in New York City – on and off-Broadway – and all over the world. The aesthetic that Seth and I developed through the years is deliberate, and at its best, invisible. In other words, the direction isn't often seen but ideally is felt. At different points in the process, we considered incorporating larger set elements, but in the end, we always tried to stage the shows simply. This was done with the help of our brilliant designers Beowulf Boritt, Aaron Copp, and others. However, the way we staged the show is just one approach. Seth and I would love to see a production like that or a production that is very different from that. We would love to see productions starring any number of actors and any type of actor (regardless of race, gender, etc.). The goal for these solo shows is to attempt to have a connection in the room with the audience. However you can make that happen, we are excited to see it.

NOTE ON TEXT

Text in [square brackets] is from the original production of *The Old Man and the Pool* and is customized to the specifics of the Broadway venue and city where it was performed. Take liberties in customizing these moments to your specific theater and city.

(A projection reads "The Old Man and the Pool." An upbeat song plays. Lights come up as **MIKE** enters.)*

MIKE. Thanks!

What better place to be at 7:30 p.m. on a Friday than right here [at the Vivian Beaumont Theater at Lincoln Center which is one of the Lincoln Centers at Lincoln Center. Congratulations on finding the correct one.]

In 2017 I went for my annual medical checkup which I always dread because I have a lot of pre-existing conditions which I call "conditions" because everything is existing if it does, and everything is "pre" unless it happened on the way to the appointment. When I see that checklist, I just circle the whole thing and I cross out "pregnant."

This year I turned forty-four and as I've gotten older, I've found that the items in the doctor's office that I thought were decorative are quite functional.

I'll give you an example. I'm at my annual checkup and my physician, this guy Doctor Walsh, says, "Blow into this tube."

It's a pulmonary test where they ask you to blow into this tube and there's a ball in the tube that simulates blowing out a candle which is why I call it "the birthday cake test" because it sort of tells you how many birthday cakes...you have left.

---

*A license to produce *The Old Man and the Pool* does not include a performance license for any third-party or copyrighted music. Licensees should create an original composition or use music in the public domain. For further information, please see the Music and Third-Party Materials Use Note on page iii.

And so, I did it. I went: *(Blowing lightly.)*

Doctor Walsh stares at the monitor attached to the machine and says, "Go ahead and do it."

But I had already done it, so I had to tell him. I said, "I did it."

And then he says, "Hm. I guess just do it again."

So now I give it a little more. I go... *(Blowing again, but harder.)*

Doctor Walsh taps on the monitor like it's a broken '80s television and he does sort of an act out. He goes, "Maybe do it more like this." *(Acting out with more physicality.)*

I thought, *I don't know a lot about breathing but I'm pretty sure it's not in the shoulders.*

Doctor Walsh says, "I don't know what to tell you, Mike, if I was just going by that machine, I'd say you're having a heart attack right now."

And when he said this, I got worried because I'm thinking, *If I thought I might be having a heart attack I would either go to the emergency room or I would call you.*

So, I said, "Am I having a heart attack?"

He said, "I don't think so."

I said, "I need a more concrete answer than that."

Doctor Walsh says, "I'm gonna send you across town to see a cardiologist for a second opinion."

I get nervous when I hear the phrase "second opinion." I was under the impression this first analysis was fact-based. I didn't know we were taking swings in the dark. If I knew it were opinion time, I'd point out that I don't enjoy sitting on paper. It makes me feel like a chicken. And I feel you could digitize some of those forms in that waiting room. I feel like I've filled a few of those out before. Those are opinions. So, I get on the crosstown bus which is sort of a slow ambulance with stops. That's another opinion. And I meet my new cardiologist Doctor Bennett and the first thing she asks me to do is... *(Stopping.)*

(To audience.) Does anybody want to guess?

(Off audience.) Yes, she says, "Blow into the tube."

I say, "No, I took that one and I got heart attack."

She says, "Oh no. That's a low score. Do you have a history of heart disease in your family?"

I said, "Actually, my dad had a heart attack when he was fifty-six and actually his dad had a heart attack when he was fifty-six so I've always thought I should just set aside that whole year, get an Airbnb by the hospital and keep a flexible schedule. I think that might be a big year for me."

Doctor Bennett says, "Well, based on your family history I would suggest doing cardio five days a week."

I said, "I don't think anybody does cardio five days a week."

She said, "A lot of people do cardio five days a week."

I said, "I don't even think professional athletes do cardio five days a week."

She says, "Professional athletes definitely do cardio five days a week."

We talk about this for about forty-five minutes. We agree to disagree. At this point I'm sweaty and out of breath. A little hungry. I'm always a little hungry.

She said, "Didn't you play sports growing up?"

I said, "Yeah, I played soccer, but I could blend in at practice. People would be like, *(Pointing one way.)*

"There's Mike!" *(Pointing the other way.)* "No, Mike's in the woods!"

And then when I was in ninth grade, I joined the wrestling team, which was a huge mistake, my teammates explained to me. In wrestling practice, you can't blend in. You have to wrestle. Or, in my case, be wrestled upon by these young muscly gentlemen whose crotches would inevitably be pressed up against my face as though they were doing a victory dance.

(Crouching down to demonstrate.)

All the while I'm wearing a women's bathing suit they call a "singlet." But I was building character. And that character was a lifeguard from the 1920s.

(Sometimes late seating is here. If so, to audience member:) Welcome to the show. You didn't miss much. A few years ago I went for my annual checkup and I failed the pulmonary test and my cardiologist said, "you should do cardio five days a week" and you're probably thinking, "Nobody does cardio five days a week" and then she said, "Didn't you play sports growing up?" and I said in high school I joined the wrestling team and that's how we got here on the floor.

(Pivot back to show.)

I hated wrestling practice so much because we had to do many pushups and at a very early age, I lost the will to push up. *(Lying on the floor.)* I'd get in that first position, and I think, *This is a nice new lying position* and then I'd sort of lean into my hands and think, *These hands are soft. These hands are nature's pillows.*

So, in practice we'd do pushups and we'd wrestle each other. I was in the 152-pound weight class and based on ability I was paired with our team's 102-pound wrestler. I don't know if you've seen a lot of 102-pound people. These are generally smaller folks. It's a little bit like wrestling your own baby. And this magical baby would pin me multiple times per practice. It was like watching a paperweight *(Miming paperweight.)* be pinned by paper. *(Miming paper pinning it.)*

So, I was terrible and of course I didn't compete but I would travel with the team and I'd wear the same outfit. If there was time permitting after the matches they would send us B-teamers out to wrestle their B-teamers. When they did this, I developed a secret strategy to be pinned as quickly as possible so this portion of my life would be over. My strategy ran into a snag when I encountered an opponent who had the same strategy. So we're out there for a while. *(Miming wrestling.)* We're flashing each other signals: *You can pin me! Here's my leg! Here's my head! I can't even do pushups! These hands are nature's pillows! Oh, I know!* It was a stalemate.

But there are three starting positions in high school wrestling that move it along. There's the "I hump you."

(Acting out "top referee" position on the floor.)

There's the "You hump me."

(Acting out "bottom referee" position on the floor.)

And then there's the "Who humps who?"

(Acting out neutral standing position.)

That's the "neutral Greco-Roman" because I believe it was the Greeks who posed the question "Who humps who?" and the Romans who answered, "Everybody." I'm not a historian. So I get into the "I hump you" with this opposing B-teamer *(Acting out top referee position.)* and the ref blows the whistle and somehow, I find myself pinning this guy. And I couldn't believe it. He couldn't believe it. My teammates were stunned. They cleared the bench. They said, "Mike, squeeze!"

(Confiding in audience.) Which in wrestling means "squeeze."

And so I *squeeeeeeze,* and all of a sudden there's blood all over the mat.

(Off audience.) No, I know. I thought, *I killed this guy. I'm gonna be on the run from the law for the rest of my life – Birbiglia the wrestling bandit. One pin, one kill. Couldn't do a pushup. Murdered a young boy with his bare hands. He called 'em "nature's pillows."*

I realize it is my own blood streaming out of my nose onto the mat based on no physical injury whatsoever. Just from the sheer nervousness of possibly winning anything at all. My body's like, *what do we do? Let's just bleed! We'll figure it out tomorrow.* Ref blows the whistle. He shouts, "Blood on the mat!" *(Pointing.)* Which was obvious. A little blood boy runs out, wipes it up with a rag, jogs off. My teammates plug my nose. They say, "Mike, you get out there and do what you just did." These fools thought I knew what I had just done. I jog back onto the mat. I get into the "I hump you." The ref blows the whistle, and I am immediately pinned. That was the closest I would ever come to winning a wrestling match for the rest of my life. And that's how I ended up here *(Pointing to stage.)* [at the Vivian Beaumont Theater at Lincoln Center]. And that's how we all ended up here in a sense.

(If there's a late person, pointing to the person:) At whatever time we chose to arrive.

So I explain all of this to my cardiologist. The bullet points. The big stuff. I said, "I don't think it's realistic that I could do cardio five days a week."

Doctor Bennett says, "What about swimming? Do you like swimming?"

   (Beat, pivot stage left.)

When I was five years old my mom took me to the YMCA pool in Worcester, Massachusetts, and I hated everything about it. It was wet. Sweaty. It smelled like... You know when you're a kid and your friend lets you smell under their cast. It's like if *that smell* became a building, and then someone fire-hosed the building with over-chlorinated water – which by way it didn't feel like they were using the proper amount of chlorine. Like, I'm not sure they read the directions. Some overzealous administrator was like, *"One pahrt water, two pahrts chlorine!"*

Everyone's like, "Janice! No!"

She's like, "I'm just doin' moy jawb!"

I don't know what the hell kind of heinous crimes they're covering up at the YMCA, but I think something may have gone down. Like there was a mob hit in the middle of the night. A buncha goons are like, *(Mafia voice.)* "Do we dig a ditch?" And then one guy's like, *(Even more Mafia-ish voice.) "Why don't we bring over da body to the YMCA? I've got a family membership. We use a guest pass for the corpse. We drop it in da pool. It disintegrates within six hours."*

It's a lot of chlorine is what I'm getting at.

And there's so much chlorine because there's so much urine. It's true. I thought that you should know this. I looked it up and it's not great out there on the Internet. I read about these scientists who analyzed a 200,000 gallon public pool and they concluded that the pool contained twenty gallons...<u>gallons</u>...of pure urine.

(Off audience.) I know. I thought this was something you should know.

Which is too much, I think. I mean, percentagewise it's not that much but if you picture it...it's a full tank of gas. It's a Ford F150 full of urine. That'll get you to [Pittsburgh].

And I feel like the good Christians of the Young Men's Christian Association are aware of the urine issue which is why there are signs everywhere begging you not to urinate in the pool. Just like, "Please don't pee our pool." Which might as well say, "What better place to pee than pool."

I'm obsessed with the signs at the Y because I feel like they tell you the stories of what has occurred at the Y. There was one that said, "Slippery when wet." You know some kids went down pretty hard on them tiles and a frazzled lifeguard grabbed a Sharpie and wrote *(Writing.)* "Slippery...when..." *(Then.)* You don't see "wet" on a lot of signage. Rarely do you see a subordinate clause in a form that values brevity. "Slippery when wet" could just say "slippery." It's wet a majority of the time. There was a sign that said, "Please shower before entering the pool." I think that was written for one guy. The first draft of that sign said, "...Greg."

But the sign I remember that was most flagrantly disobeyed at the YMCA was in the locker room and it said, "Please remain properly covered." I never witnessed that. When I was five my mom took me into the women's locker room, and I had never seen a vagina before and then I saw 100 vaginas. When I was six, she sent me into the men's locker room and the only thing more shocking than 100 vaginas is 100 penises at eye level. And they were grown-up penises, which is a surprisingly crucial detail because I just had the six-year-old penis and I'm looking at these grown-up penises thinking, *Oh no. This is gonna be a long life.* So now I'm looking side to side for child penises – please don't quote this out of context. We could end a career with a few sloppy keystrokes.

I remember that locker room so well because when I was seven there was this old man who would come to the locker room every day. Probably the oldest man I'd ever seen. Must have been 120...130 years old and he'd sit on the bench 100% naked.

(Sitting on stool as the old man.)

He was not properly covered. It's possible he had been peeing in that pool all day. And this ancient man would massage his testicles with baby powder... *(Confiding in audience.)* Stay with me.

To be clear I'm not being intentionally gratuitous. I'm relaying an accurate memory from my childhood that I feel might be humorous if it was part of your memory also.

(Returning to the position of the old man on the stool.)

The key thing about this old man is that he would really take his time. Like a resin bag on a pitcher's mound. So much patience. So much powder.

(Standing up, walking downstage left.)

So I don't know if it was the blinding combination of chlorine and urine or the jungle of eye-level genitalia or the 175-year-old man desperately trying to ease the friction between his scrotum and his inner thigh but I remember thinking, *I will never return to the YMCA Pool.*

(Beat.)

So I explain this to my cardiologist. At this point it was nightfall. We were roasting marshmallows over a burning file cabinet.

I said, "I don't want to get into the details, but I actually do not enjoy swimming."

Doctor Bennett said, "Mike, you might want to reconsider that position. It's a great sport for people your age. Good for increasing lung capacity, easy on the joints."

Then she said, "Do you happen to live near a YMCA pool?"

I said, "I do. I live a short walk from the Brooklyn YMCA but it's just not my thing."

She said, "I think it might be for the best if you spent some time at the YMCA pool."

I said, "I think I'm not gonna do what's for the best."

That night I'm riding the subway home to Brooklyn.

(Walking with stool, placing stage right.)

And I'm experiencing this shortness of breath that I sometimes get from anxiety. I've had this since I was a kid. Where I feel like I can't catch...my breath. And sometimes it's so bad I'm convinced I'm going to pass out. I remember when I was a kid riding in the car with my dad and I'm short of breath my dad said, "Why are you breathing like that?" Which is always helpful when you're experiencing a physical difficulty for a person in authority to scold you until it goes away.

I'm on the subway and I'm thinking about my grandfather. My father's dad worked in the subway tunnels as an electrician in the '30s. He was an electrician. And in the '30s, they would blow up dynamite in these tunnels, and they'd send the electricians in. They'd be the first ones in to light up these dark, dark tunnels. It's a very dangerous job. After that he worked at a bodega in Bushwick and supposedly one of his regulars came in and said, "How's it going, Joe?" And he just keeled over the counter and died. Which is sad...but it's also a pretty funny response if you think about it. In some ways he was the original comedian in the family. That's an extraordinary level of commitment.

But I think about him a lot. I never met my grandfather, but I wish I had. And then when I was nineteen years old, I'm in my college dorm and I get a call from my mom and she said, "Dad collapsed on the living room floor." He had a heart attack. She said, "I called 9-1-1 and the ambulance rushed him to Mass General Hospital." And I get off the phone with my mom and tell my roommate Danny and you know how sometimes you think you're okay until you relay the same piece of information to someone else and mid-sentence your voice collapses into tears? I borrowed a friend's car and drove 400 miles to Boston and saw my dad in the hospital bed. They had performed an emergency angioplasty that saved his life. They inserted a metal stent in one of his coronary arteries, but he's all beat up, bandages around his chest and the electrodes under his rib cage.

I feel like we don't choose what we remember from our own lives but what I remember the most about that day is that it was the first time I saw my dad as a person. And the second thing I remember is that when I left visiting hours I didn't say "I love you" to my dad. I wanted to.

We're not an I love you family. We say, "Take care."

(To audience member.) It's okay for you to laugh because it's not the same. At all. Like it's not even that similar. "Take care" is an odd substitution for "I love you" for two reasons.

   (Beat.)

First of all, it doesn't have the word "love" in it. Second of all, it's sort of a passive aggressive command as if to say, "I'm gonna need you to do something for me. Take care." You know what I mean? And I've tried to reverse the cycle in subtle ways. A few years ago I called my mom for Mother's Day, and I said, "Mom...I really appreciate you." There was silence on the other end of the phone for a few moments and then she said, "Bye now."

So I get off at my subway stop in Brooklyn and I walk home to my wife Jenny and our daughter Oona who was three years old at the time. When you have a child that young you know that your apartment becomes what would happen if you had a rave at a bakery. Sparkles and glow sticks and bubble-makers and everybody's like, "Do you have water?" All kinds of arts and crafts. We paint all over the walls because it's a rental. So there's dinosaurs and people. It's like a creationism museum. That day Jenny and Oona were making these beaded bracelets and Oona made me this one.

(Holding up beaded bracelet on left wrist.)

She says, "Dad, it says silly. It's to remind you to be silly."

I thought, *Thank God. I do sometimes need the reminder.*

Then Jenny pulls me aside. She says, "Mo..." (She calls me Mo and I call her Clo; there's no real story.)

She says, "Mo, how did it go at the doctor?

I say, "Well, the pulmonary test said I was having a heart attack but the doctor said he didn't think I was so... *(Miming weighing the balance.)* ...not great."

So Jenny's worried and because she's worried, I'm worried. We're sort of an anxious improv group. I initiate with a worry and she "yes ands" the worry with some misgivings and then I close out the scene with some neuroses and then sometimes we have sex which is so fun.

That night I'm reading Oona a book about penguins and when I'm with Oona my anxiety melts away because she's silly. Like the bracelet. She goes, "Dad, you have yellow teeth."

I said, "Yeah, I try not to think about it too much."

Then she picks up her cat puppet named "Meow Meow" and Meow Meow says, *"Those are the yellowest teeth I've ever seen."*

And now I'm trying <u>not</u> to laugh because I love that Oona's funny, but I don't want her to be an insult comic and a ventriloquist.

So then I'm trying to out-silly Oona. I make up a joke about penguins. I say, "What does the penguin say to her parents when she's hungry?"

Oona said, "What?"

I said, "Waddle we have for dinner?"

(*Off audience.*)

Don't feel like you have to laugh at that joke. It's not *for you.* I write some jokes *for you,* and I write some jokes *for my daughter.* What you need to know for the story is that it killed. Oona was like, *"Ha! Waddle we have for dinnah?!"*

Because kids love puns and all toddlers sort of have a Boston accent. They're like *"I'm tie-ahd"* and Boston toddlers are like, *"I'm wicked tie-ahd."*

So we're reading the penguin book and I say, "Mom's gonna brush your hair in a minute."

And she says, "She's not yowa mom, she's moy mom."

I said, "That's what my therapist keeps telling me."

(*Aside to the audience.*) *You* liked that joke, but *she* didn't like that one so everybody gets their own jokes which is fun.

I do think there's some truth to that joke. Some people say we project onto our partner the quality in our parent who was hardest on us, and I don't think it's entirely true. I think the reason I married my dad is that he loves me and sometimes I wonder why because I'm a bad boy.

So Jenny walks in to brush Oona's hair and says, "Do you smell that?"

I said, "Which thing?"

Jenny says, "Mildew."

I said, "I can't smell mildew because I'm from Massachusetts which is a state that's made of mildew."

But she's worried about it. Jenny says, "I don't think Oona can sleep in her bedroom until we get the mildew situation figured out."

I say, "It's okay. Until we get the mildew resolved I'll sleep in Oona's bed and Oona can sleep in our bed."

And to make me feel better about this Jenny and Oona started calling me "Mildew Man."

So an hour later mildew man is lying in his daughter's mildew-scented bed alone and I'm writing in my journal. I like to write in my journal every few nights because if you write down what you're saddest about or angriest about you can start to see your own life as a story. When you see your own life as a story, sometimes you can zoom out and encourage the main character to make better decisions.

That night I wrote in my journal: "My dad had a heart attack when he was fifty-six and his dad had a heart attack when he was fifty-six. And today I realized...

"When I turn fifty-six, Oona will be nineteen."

> *(Optional Projection Cue: The words "When I turn fifty-six, Oona will be nineteen," written in **MIKE**'s handwriting, appear across the screen as **MIKE** delivers the line.)*

The next morning, I woke up and I walked to the Brooklyn YMCA.

> *(Walking stage right, placing stool in vom.)*

I didn't need directions. *(Sniffing air.)* I just followed that chlorine smell. I approached the swim desk and asked to speak with the director of aquatics.

They introduced me to a woman named Vanessa and I said, "Vanessa, I'd like to take a swim lesson if possible."

She said, "I'd have to come down to the pool and evaluate your level."

I said, "No need. Just write down zero or negative twenty or drowning or dead. Whatever the lowest is."

She said, "I'd have to see it for myself."

I said, "Is it a fetish thing? Because I could do sort of a dry act-out here at the desk."

I walk into the locker room, and I put on my swim trunks. I've never worn a Speedo. I wear sort of a "Speed-less." It's bunchy and always damp even fresh out of the dryer. I meet Vanessa down at the pool and the first thing she says to me is, "Where's your swim cap?"

I say, "I don't have a swim cap."

She says, "It's mandatory unless you're completely bald."

I say, "I don't like how you leaned on the word 'completely.' I'm not even remotely bald."

Vanessa says, "You can borrow my extra swim cap."

She hands me her swim cap which is considerably smaller than my head. So I squeeze Vanessa's tiny swim cap onto my head and Vanessa says, "Hop in the instructional lane and show me your stuff." (*Pointing to pool area.*)

At this point I feel like I've made it clear that I don't have stuff. I don't have a repertoire. But I get in the instructional lane, and I'm giving it all I got. (*Thrashing with arms.*) I may have been swimming towards the bottom. I looked like what would happen if you dropped a blender in a pool. I'm blending the water into a chlorine smoothie.

By the way, "the instructional lane" is also "the walkers' lane." (*Pointing out the separate lanes while mimicking the walkers.*) So as I'm blending there are these aggressive, elderly walkers blowing past me. I think one of them tried to dunk my head. *(Dunking motion.)* And it's packed. *(Crowded pool physicality.)* Only in this city is there traffic in the pool.

I say, "Vanessa, is it always this crowded?"

She says, "No, it's the springtime. Everyone's getting ready for summer!"

I say, "Oh, they want a body like this." *(Pointing to own body.)*

It was a joke. It wasn't a stage-worthy joke. Nothing that I would share with you here [at the Vivian Beaumont Theater]. It was a conversational piece of witty repartee intended to forge a human bond between myself and my new swim instructor.

She didn't hear it.

She said, "What?" *(Shouting, to indicate that Vanessa is far away.)*

I said, "Nothing." *(Not shouting.)*

She said, "Mike! I can't hear you. You have to shout!"

I say, *(Hesitating, beat.)* "VANESSA...THEY WANT A BODY...LIKE THIS!"

A joke without proper context or softness of cadence or comedic delivery is often a statement of pure insanity. Because all two hundred members of the pool simultaneously swiveled their heads to see the body attached to this flamboyantly confident voice.

I don't have "a swimmer's body." I have sort of "a drowner's body," where it looks like I'm drowning at all times even when I'm not near water. Even shirtless and dry, people are like, "Are you OK?" It's sort of a "river corpse body."

So I'm blending water for about ninety seconds *(Blending water.)* until I'm convinced I'm on the verge of my own death and then I stand up.

(Standing up, indicating water level.)

It's about four feet of water.

Then I get out of the pool and dry myself off with fifteen or twenty of those dish rag-size YMCA towels. I even put one under each foot because Vanessa explains that there can be fungus in the puddles. I'm thinking, *This place is a death trap. I gotta get the hell outta here. I came in for some cardio and now I am mainlining spores.*

I walk over to the aquatics desk and say, "Vanessa, now that you've evaluated my level, can we possibly arrange a swim lesson?"

Vanessa says, "I just don't have time for that in my schedule." Which means that I had auditioned for swim lessons and I didn't get the part.

Vanessa feels bad for me and she says, "Look, Mike, If you come in Wednesday at 8 a.m. I can probably squeeze you in for twenty minutes, but if you want to take this seriously, I would recommend you swim *on your own* five days a week."

I said, "I don't think anybody swims five days a week."

She said, "A lot of people swim five days a week."

I said, "I don't even think Michael Phelps swims five days a week."

She said, "Michael Phelps definitely swims five days a week."

We talk about this for forty-five minutes. We agree to disagree.

I start swimming one day a week. I got into it. I got my own YMCA swim cap. I got those goggles that have a lifetime guarantee not to fit your face once ever. I got a lock for my locker and flip flops for the fungus puddles. I got a swim bag with a side pocket for wet bathing suits and fresh produce. Every Wednesday at 8 a.m. I'd swim with Vanessa and then afterwards I'd go to this juice place on the corner and get a big juice the size of a horse bucket and I remember thinking, *This is who I am now. I swim. I juice. I'm juicy! I should get some of those pants that say "juicy" on the ass because that's sort of my deal now and everybody gets it.*

My favorite part about swimming is that no matter how bad you are at swimming...

> *(Optional Projection Cue: Rippling water appears behind* **MIKE***.)*

...when you swim underwater, and you kick off the wall for those few moments you feel like you're an underwater explorer or someone who knows how to swim. And then your body floats towards the top because the human body has neutral buoyancy. I love how when you're in the pool there are no phones or emails or calendars. In some ways there's no time. I love that sometimes in life everything feels so heavy but when you're underwater it feels so light. Sometimes everything in your life is so loud but when you're underwater it's so quiet. Sometimes you can even hear yourself think. One day I remember thinking: *I'm so lucky to be alive.*

> *(Cue: End water projection.)*

So for six months I swim one day a week and then one day there's a torrential downpour in Brooklyn. And it's so bad it's raining in our kitchen. I don't know if you've been in a kitchen, but the weather is generally mild. It almost never rains in kitchens. So I call my friend who's in construction and I said "Is it safe to live in this building?" It's this 100-year-old apartment building. And she came over and walks up onto the roof and said, "There are holes on the roof of the building and on the side of the building."

And then she comes inside the apartment and walks into Oona's bedroom and she says, "I think that might be mold." So we have it tested and it turns out we have black mold which is the dangerous kind tied to asthma and all kinds of problems. They said, "We would recommend you move out immediately until this is resolved."

So we move into an Airbnb, which by the way, no breakfast. Which is *one of the letters*. I don't mean to nitpick but it's a wildly misleading acronym. It's like if you showed up at an AA meeting and they were like, "We're livestreaming." And you're like, "I had heard it was sort of a private thing." They're like, "Pop open a wine cooler. We're gonna dish some goss!"

I had found this Airbnb. I have sort of an obsessive personality. If you don't know someone who's obsessive, all you need to know is that it's a very sexy quality. Your husband will disappear down an Airbnb rabbit hole for seven hours and when he comes up for air, he'll eat a whole box of Triscuits and you'll think, *I wanna bang this guy.*

The apartment was sort of a debacle. It didn't look anything like the photos. It's almost like they used one of those special lenses where it photographs *(Gesticulating from stage left to stage right.)* a different apartment.

And there was no thermostat. There was heat but there was no way to indicate how much heat you thought might be a good amount of heat if you wanted to stay alive. It's three in the morning and it's ninety degrees. Jenny and Oona and I are all awake and I'm desperate. I'm wandering around this Airbnb trying to find some way to change the temperature. Around three a.m. I find a communal thermostat for the entire building in the back of the lobby padlocked behind this plexiglass encasement. And this is nothing like anything I've ever done in my life but I hulk-smashed the glass and changed the thermostat to zero and saved my family's lives.

But the point of the story is that the next morning I overslept and I missed my swim lesson with Vanessa for the first time and then the next week I didn't go to my swim lesson again because it was so fun not going the first time. And then I just stopped swimming.

I think about this a lot, in a general sense: *Why do we stop doing the thing we know we should be doing?*

And for me I prioritize things that will keep me alive in the short term over things that will keep me alive in the long term because if I'm not alive in the short term I definitely won't be alive in the long term.

So I stopped swimming but I still had the appetite of someone who swims, which is to say I was eating quite a bit. And I was juicing. I went for my annual checkup and Doctor Walsh asks me to step on the scale and they still have that old fashioned abacus thing.

> *(Pantomiming measuring weight on an old-fashioned doctor's scale, sometimes called a "beam scale." The pantomiming goes from wide to narrow as the doctor gets closer to the correct weight.)*

He's like, "You're not 1000 pounds, you're not zero pounds you're not 970 pounds, you're not 22 pounds, you're not 740 pounds, you're not 111 pounds."

I'm like, *What time is it?*

> *(Looking at watch, same "balancing physicality" except with wrist motions.)*

He's like, "It's not two o'clock, it's not six o'clock. it's not 2:45, it's not 3:15..."

Doctor Walsh was worried about my weight. He said, "You've gained a lot of weight in the last year."

I said, "That's surprising because I've been swimming as well as juicing."

Doctor Walsh took my blood and then I took his because it was sort of like a sleepover theme.

A week later I'm at a hotel in Columbus, Ohio, and Doctor Walsh calls me and he says, "I got your blood results back and your bad cholesterol is bad..."

I said, "That lines up."

He said, "Your good cholesterol is bad..."

I said, "Nobody's perfect."

Then he said, "You have type two diabetes."

　　(Beat.)

When he told me this, I got that shortness of breath I told you about earlier but there are several times in my live I've gotten it to an extreme.

　　(Beat.)

When I was twenty, I was driving home from my college for Christmas break and I pulled over at a rest stop to pee and there was blood in my pee. I had never seen blood that looks like this. The moment it would hit the water it would explode like fireworks. *Poof! Poof! Congratulations! (Pantomiming fireworks.)* And I was so anxious I sped home and woke up my parents. My dad is a doctor and my mom is a nurse so they know that bloody fireworks are not a great sign. So the next morning my dad takes me to a urologist friend of his and the urologist asks me to take my pants down and while he's looking around, I start to chime in with my own theories which I find doctors enjoy that: when you view the medical visit as sort of a *collab.*

I said to my urologist, and I can never un-say this. I said, "Is it possible that the blood is from me masturbating too often?"

So that's something I said, out loud... *(To audience center, shouting.)* to my dad's friend.

I have to say – based on his reaction – if a urology drinking game does exist, I think that might be the phrase that pays. Because he looked entirely unfazed by this question. He said, "No, it's not it" and then he pounded a tumbler of whiskey from behind his desk.

He said, "But I'm worried about the blood, I'm gonna have you come into the hospital tomorrow morning and put you under anesthesia for a cystoscopy." I didn't know what that meant. It's where they take a camera and they stick it through your penis to look into your bladder. You're probably thinking, *Mike, a camera can't fit through a penis.*

Good news and bad news on that front.

The good news is that it can and the bad news is the same.

The next morning at five a.m. I wake up and my mom drives me to the hospital and I'm lying in the surgical gurney and I'm wearing the cloth smock and I'm shivering.

(Lying on the stage.) The nurse puts the IV in and I fall asleep. And I have to say – even shivering, on drugs, at a hospital. I still always enjoy a nice nap.

While I'm under, the doctor finds something in my bladder and he decided to keep me under and take it out. So as I'm coming to *(Sitting up.)* the doctor explains that they found something in my bladder. It could be cancer. They don't know and they're gonna do a biopsy on it and they should know in a few days. So from December 22, 1999, until December 27, 1999, I just thought the worst.

> *(Note: The year can vary in relation to when
> the actor was around twenty-one years old.)*

I just thought, *I'm gonna die.* And I walked into my bedroom in my parents' house and I had the shortness of breath to an extreme I had never felt where I felt like I couldn't really talk. I didn't talk to my family. I didn't call my friends... *(Confiding to audience.)* And I'm someone who talks quite a bit. I mean, I gathered you here tonight. But when I thought that I might die it silenced me.

(Beat.)

A few days later the biopsy comes back and it turns out they had taken out a malignant tumor from my bladder but I was lucky because they caught it early enough so they decided not to do chemo or radiation because they thought maybe it was an anomaly and maybe it was because every year I go for a cystoscopy and it hasn't come back.

So when Doctor Walsh tells me that I have diabetes it flashes me back to this moment. Not because cancer and diabetes are the same but they're both co-morbidities and the thing about co-morbidities is that sometimes they team up to form a single morbidity. *(Miming dribbling.)* It's cancer to diabetes, diabetes to heart disease. Heart disease scores! And then they all high five...and then I'm dead.

When Doctor Walsh told me I had type two diabetes I was walking from my hotel room in Columbus Ohio to the front desk of the hotel to pick up a pizza I had ordered for delivery. Which I'm not proud of. I have terrible habits. For starters, *this* is my job. I'm up here onstage usually in cities where I don't live.

(Crossing to one side of the stage.)

I work up an appetite walking over here. Sometimes I go over here.

(Crossing to the other side of the stage.)

Sometimes I pretend to wrestle.

Typically, I get back to my hotel at eleven o'clock at night. And the thing about healthy food is that it goes to bed early. Healthy food's like: *I'm heading in for the night! I have a big morning providing nutrients.* Unhealthy food is like, *I'm gonna hang. I saw a microwave on the corner, I might pop in and see what happens.*

Pizza stays up all night. Pizza loves to party. And I love pizza. My problem with pizza is that when I see a pizza I can only view it as a single serving and more often than not it was designed for a group. And I'm physically drawn to it. It's almost sexual. I wouldn't have sex with pizza but if I ate a pizza alone, I wouldn't mention it to my wife. Does that make sense? I love pizza so much I get excited when I see the word "plaza," because the word "pizza" itself is exciting. It's got pizza slices in it. Each of the Zs is two slices. The "A" is a slice. It's five slices in one word which is a rarely used literary device I invented called "onomatopizza."

Doctor Walsh makes a series of recommendations. He says, "I'd like to put you on a statin for your cholesterol and a diabetes medication."

I said, "I'd prefer to deal with this without medication because I'm a doctor also." I said, "I'd prefer to try to lose weight on my own and see if I can reverse the diabetes."

He said, "I'm not optimistic." He said, "It would have to be so drastic. You'd have to cut sugar, fries..."

And then I start thinking about "sugar fries" which isn't technically a food but then I start thinking *maybe it should be a food.* It's a beautiful combination of ingredients. There's an obvious theme song *(Singing.)* "Sugar fries, sugar fries, shug – shug – sugar fries, sugar fries in my eyes!"

Doctor Walsh said, "Are you listening to me?"

I said, "Obviously I'm listening to you but I am also listening to the song I just wrote in my head about vegetables." I thought it was too early to spring the sugar fries concept on him.

The next morning I fly home and Jenny and I take Oona for her first swim lesson and after the lesson they let the grown-ups get in the shallow end with the kids and Oona says "Dad, let's talk under-watah!"

And I say, "Okay!"

I go underwater and all I hear is, "Blah blah blah blah."

When I come up for air she says, "What did I say?"

I said, "I don't know."

She said, "I love you, Dad."

I said, "I love you too, Oona."

That night we're lying in bed reading this book about the days of the week and sometimes when Oona doesn't know a new word yet she just says a different word so instead of "days of the week" she said, "the days of us." And I thought, *that's better.*

That night I'm lying in bed and I'm thinking about what my doctor said to me and I'm experiencing the shortness of breath and I write in my journal: "I think I may die soon."

> *(Optional Projection Cue: The words "I think I may die soon," written in* **MIKE**'s *handwriting, appear across the screen.)*

The next morning I get a phone call from my mom. She said, "Dad had another heart attack." But he was okay. I guess he's getting the hang of heart attacks. He was working at the hospital, felt it coming on, and walked into the emergency room. He sort of pointed to his chest and said, "Hey." I'm not sure what he said. But it was like a fireman walking into the station and saying, "I'm on fire. We all know what to do!"

I said, *(On phone.)* "Mom, should I come home?

She said, *(On phone.)* "He's doing okay and you're coming home next week for Christmas."

So a week later I'm driving Jenny and Oona home for Christmas and it's always sort of involved with family gatherings because Jenny is an introvert and I'm an extrovert. An extrovert is someone who gets energy from being around other people and an introvert doesn't like you. Or she might like you but she's gonna need me to explain why we're leaving. And it's Christmas and Jenny's Jewish so I always have to explain that there's this guy, and he was born in a barn, which usually flies under the radar, but this one went wide. Kings showed up. And wise men. Although they were Jewish, so it could have been "the Weissmans." So it was the Kings and the Weissmans and they're kvetching and kvelling and I don't know why. "It's not God!" And I'm no kind of authority on any of this although I have gotten more interested in Jesus as I've gotten older, which is why I brought you here tonight. There's a pamphlet under your seat...

And our family doesn't do a very religious Christmas. If anything the theme is chicken parmesan. We eat so much of it. But that year it was a charged subject because my dad had just had a heart attack and we're sitting at the dining room table and there's chicken parmesan and ziti and garlic bread which are all basically the same food in different shapes.

My dad says: "Michael, please pass the chicken parmesan."

My dad just had a heart attack and he's already had a serving of chicken parmesan. And so I pick up the plate of chicken parmesan but I'm not passing it because it feels almost like I'm holding a bowl full of guns. And I can feel tension rising and finally I say, "Vince..." We call my dad Vince. I go, "Vince... That's enough chicken parmesan."

Which I'm pretty sure is a deleted scene from *The Godfather*.

Vince had the perfect response.

He says, "Michael, I want to talk to you about your type two diabetes."

I say, "I'm working on it. I'm trying to change my diet like you are."

Then my brother Joe says, "You know Mike, you should write a will."

I thought, *How did we get here?*

You have to be really close with someone when you tell them you have a disease for their response to be "I'd love to have some of your stuff."

That night we're saying goodbye to my parents at the front door and I have a fear that when I'm saying goodbye to my dad, it might be "goodbye."

So I say, "Mom...Dad...take care."

I don't know why it's so hard for me to say I love you to my parents but it is.

Sometimes I feel like we get so close to it. A few years ago a friend of ours died and I called my mom and I said, "I'm so sorry about John Harding."

And she said, "We were lucky because when he called us last week, he knew it would be the last time we'd get to speak and so we were able to tell him we loved him."

    (Beat.)

And I thought, *Oh wow. I've cracked the code. All you need is the approximate date of your own death. You just need a literal deadline.*

I'm thinking about all of this late that night as we're driving home. Oona's asleep in the backseat and I said to my wife, "Clo, do you think we should write a will?" And she doesn't respond.

Jen and I don't have this in common. When someone asks me a question, I feel a social responsibility to reply but Jen doesn't have that. She ghosted me in person.

So I take matters into my own hands and I call this lawyer who writes wills. We'll call him "Will." And Will comes over to our apartment and I'm sitting with Jenny and Will at our kitchen table, and it gets very serious right away. He says, "What happens if Mike gets hit by a bus?"

I said, "Um…Jen…gets the money?"

He says, "What if you and Jen get hit by the same bus?"

I said, "Um…our daughter Oona gets the money."

Will said, "Who's in charge of Oona?"

I said, "The bus driver?"

Then it was silent for about forty minutes.

Of course, you really can get hit by the bus. It's not an outrageous scenario. A few years ago I was in the back of an Uber [here] and the driver made a left turn onto a bridge and hits a pedestrian. She was okay but she went down hard and then she popped up and said, *(Arms up.)* "I'm good!" Because [New Yorkers] are resilient. And often drunk. But it was shocking. The first thing I thought was *(Typing in phone.)* One star.

I mean…there are an infinite number of ways any of us can die.

I read about a woman who died from a coconut falling on her head. Which is the ultimate example of she did not see that coming. And my question is, with all due respect if you know someone who was killed by a coconut…should we eat the coconut? I mean…it's ripe.

I read about a guy who died in a cockroach eating competition. No, I know...*which part of Florida was it in?* Deerfield Beach. It doesn't matter.

The point is we're sitting with Will and we're filling out what's called a "death questionnaire," and the first few questions are easy.

Name...*alright. (Sitting on stool, pantomiming signature.)*

Email: Come on!

Date you were married: We can look that up!

Will says, "I'm gonna go, but I'll leave the death questionnaire here on the kitchen table and if you get it back to me in a few days we can get this finished."

And the death questionnaire sits on our kitchen table for a week.

And then a month.

And then three years.

That's how much Jenny and I don't want to discuss death.

But we have to talk about it. I mean at that point, Oona was six. When I was six my grandparents died, the Challenger exploded. I grew up in the '80s. That happened live on television at school. My teacher rolled the TV into class *(Pantomiming rolling TV.)* and said, "Today we will see seven brave astronauts going to space."

"Actually..." *(Rolling other way.)* "We're gonna watch *The Sound of Music.*"

We were six. We were like *"AHHHH. Where did they go?!"*

And I went to Catholic school so the teachers said, "They're in a better place." I was like, *Better than space? I don't know.*

That's what all the grown-ups said when someone died. "They're in a better place." And I always took solace in that but as I got older, I began to feel like people telling me that were not as confident as I had originally thought.

When I was twenty-one a close friend of our family passed away. Mister Naples. He was like a second father to me. He was at every Christmas Parmesan. When my parents would go on vacation Joe and I would stay at his house and we loved it because he was funny and he was the first person in my life who would let us in on grownup jokes and he was sort of rich. When you rang his doorbell, it wouldn't go "ding dong." *(Waving arms and torso back in forth in an exaggerated pantomime of long chime doorbell.)* It would go, "Bing bong bing bong bing bong bing bong!" and we were like, "This dude is rich. That's how you spend money right there. You get yourself a good doorbell game."

When Mister Naples was fifty-eight, he died suddenly. It was devastating. We're all crying our eyes out at the church. And I'm looking at Mr. Naples' body and it's embalmed. I don't think I'd seen a body embalmed up close. I'm thinking, *Is this the best plan. Do we really need one last facial?* Can we be honest about the embalming thing? The people don't look good. They look puffy. If we're going to manipulate the body, why not taxidermy? Like, *it's so sad about Mister Naples, but he's catchin' that football!* Something with a little energy. Let's give him a win on the way out!

What I remember most about that day is that after the funeral we get to our friend's house and everyone starts drinking. And I remember it so well because my parents don't really drink. A few hours later I'm thinking we're gonna go home and my parents keep drinking. An hour later they're drunk. They're slurring their words and spitting as they talk and making no sense and it was the first time it hit me: I don't know if anyone can handle death.

(Beat.)

Jenny and I never wrote a will but I did start to see a nutritionist which isn't the same thing at all but is a positive step.

If you haven't gone to a nutritionist, you're not missing too much. They know the same stuff as us. Imagine your most annoying friend...and then imagine if that person charged you. She's like, "You know what's healthy? Vegetables." I'm like, *I had heard that from everyone. Have you been talking to everyone?*

But she was very encouraging. Her name is Christina and she got very granular right away. She said, "How soft are your stools?"

I said, "I don't have a point of comparison. Softer than a dog, harder than a pigeon?" I didn't know we were supposed to keep track. Did I miss a meeting? I worry about people who have a really good answer, like – DELICATE! You're like, "Eeee." *(Cringing.)*

Christina says, "Do you have any pre-existing conditions?"

I said, "I had bladder cancer, I have type two diabetes, I eat sugar fries."

Then Christina says, "When do you have your best night's sleep?"

I say, "When I read." Because when I read my brain is like, *I'm out. I was under the impression there's a film adaptation. I had no idea what I was getting into.*

So it got me in the habit of reading before bed. But I would find that I would read and then I'd fall asleep and then my lamp would still be on so I got this app on my phone called Wemo. It's a timer that shuts off your bedside lamp or whatever is plugged into the wall after fifteen or twenty minutes. So I'd set my Wemo, take my sleep medication, get in my sleeping bag, and then I read my book, and then while I was asleep the lights would go... *(Making the lamp clicking noise.)*

But one night I didn't fall asleep. I set my Wemo. I get in my sleeping bag. I take my sleeping medication and I'm reading the book and I'm completely absorbed in the characters and the story – and then as the plot is reaching its climax...

> *(Walking downstage, making lamp clicking noise.)*

And in some way, it was the closest I've come to experiencing my own death. And I start thinking, Wemo could market themselves as a death simulator. And they could call it "WeDie." Or "WeNoMo."

So now I'm doing WeNoMo. I'm seeing a nutritionist. I'm monitoring my stools. And I start thinking about this quote that has stuck with me for a long time. About twenty years ago I was watching the great musician Warren Zevon as a guest on the David Letterman Show and he was dying of terminal lung cancer. It was very sad and he knew it. And Letterman asked him, "Experiencing this the way you are...what can you teach us about life and death?"

And Warren Zevon said, "Enjoy every sandwich."

I think for the year I started to see a nutritionist I think I started to enjoy every sandwich. When I would eat, I would just eat and I would still eat pizza but I wouldn't eat the whole pie. I'd just have one or two slices. In some way I enjoyed it more. This idea that I could sip the nectar of the gods without downing the whole jug. After about a year of this, I went for my annual checkup and Doctor Walsh took my blood and I met with him a few days later and he says, "You know Mike, I'm surprised to report you've actually reversed your type two diabetes...but I want you to blow into this tube."

And I so did. *(Blowing.)*

And he said, "Do it again."

And I did. *(Blowing.)*

And then he said, "Mike, let me show you something." He brings me over to his computer screen. "When a healthy person your age blows into that tube the line goes a little bit like this..."

> *(Optional Projection Cue: A graph appears behind* **MIKE**, *one-by-one showing three sample spirometry test results. If a projection is not helpful, physicalize the upward and downward motion of the graph.)*

> *(Pointing to screen, a projection where the line goes up and then across.)*

"When someone with obstructed breathing blows into the tube it looks like this:"

> *(Pointing to screen, a projection where the line goes up, and then across, and then down.)*

"When you do it, the line goes like this:"

> *(Pointing to screen, a projection where the line goes quickly up then down.)*

He says, "I don't know what to tell you, Mike. Because in the short term there's not much we can do. I've sent you to a cardiologist. But in the long term with your history of heart disease, bladder cancer, and diabetes this just isn't ideal."

> *(Walking downstage center.)*

I had never heard my doctor sound so worried but have no plan. And that night I'm lying in bed with Oona that night after she's fallen asleep and I'm experiencing that shortness of breath except this time I'm thinking about how I'll be thinking about my breathing for the rest of my life. The same way that since I was twenty years old, I think about the color of the water in the toilet every time I pee. The same way since I was twenty that every night before I fall asleep I have this sinking fear that I might hurt myself in my sleep.

And I pick up my journal and I open it up, and I can't write anything.

The next morning I wake up and walk to the Brooklyn YMCA and I start swimming five days a week.

You're probably thinking, *Nobody swims five days a week.*

I'm telling you, "I swim five days a week."

You're probably thinking, *Michael Phelps doesn't swim five days a week.* I'm telling you, "Michael Phelps and I, both individually and at the same level, swim five days a week."

And I pick up this book on breathing called *Breath*. It's an elementary start. And I started doing this exercise where you hold your breath for increasingly long increments of time which is a technique employed by yoga teachers and middle school bullies. I would practice this underwater at the YMCA. *(Pantomiming swimming underwater center stage.)* One day, I'm swimming underwater two thirds the length of one lane and when I surface, I see a sign I had never noticed.

It says, "No breath holding."

I thought, *That's so odd.* So I go, "Vanessa, what does that mean? No breath holding?"

Vanessa said, "Last summer there were these two guys taking turns holding their breath as a competition and then one of them died."

> *(Beat,* **MIKE** *is surprised by interrupting audience laughter.)*

Oh, I'm sorry. I'm just gonna stop you right there. I think the appropriate thing to do right now would be to have a moment of silence for this man who died holding his breath in the YMCA pool.

(Usually laughter.)

Okay, I'm actually gonna stop the show here for a moment.

> *(Standing up. This final portion of the show is a semi-improvised exercise in convincing the audience not to laugh when, typically, they laugh harder. The text below is flexible based on how much the audience is reacting. The game of this scene is that the more serious the performer is, the more the audience will laugh.)*

So I know we joked about a lot of dark topics earlier, but I thought with this one we would just sort of give it some space and have a moment of silence for this man who died holding his breath in the YMCA pool. Can you help me with that?

(Usually laughter.)

Actually, I'm gonna stop you right there. *(To a specific person.)* I don't want to single anyone out... Can we turn on the house lights?

(House lights turn on.)

(To audience member.) We're doing something over here right now. We're having a moment of silence for a man who died in the YMCA pool and you're doing something different. So if you could just be more respectful of this man who died...holding his breath...

(To another audience member who's laughing.) Okay you're not helping. You know who's not laughing right

now. Do you know who's not laughing right now? This man who died holding his breath in the YMCA pool.

Look, I know that earlier I had some jokes about my own cancer and diabetes and writing my own will. That stuff was funny. But this is different. We're talking about a man who died holding his breath in the YMCA pool.

(Usually a laugh. Then, to the mezzanine.) Maybe folks are in from out of town. I don't know how they do things where you come from but here in [New York City] in every comedy show there are the portions of the show where we laugh and a portion of the show where we have a moment of silence for a man who died holding his breath in the YMCA pool. If you're not mature enough to handle that maybe you should go.

(Usually a laugh, then, to a specific audience member.) Is that your sense of humor? You think that's funny? When you're feeling down and you need a pick me up you think of a man who died holding his breath in the YMCA pool??

> *(Usually a laugh, then, ending the semi-improvised section and addressing the entire audience.)*

Okay, we're gonna try something different. We're gonna have a hard restart. I think as a group we can really focus and give this man a moment of silence. I believe we can do this. Let's take a deep breath...

> *(Breathing in, audience breathing in.)*

Not too long!

> *(Then.)*

If there's one thing we learned from this man who died holding his breath it is to be judicious with the length of one's breath, when holding one's breath.

Okay, let me try one last thing. I really believe we can do this. It's a good group of people. If you could just repeat after me:

We're going to have a a moment of silence.

 (Repeated by audience.)

For this man who died...

 (Repeated by audience.)

Holding his breath...

 (Repeated by audience.)

In the YMCA pool...

 (Repeated by audience.)

Once we achieve...

 (Repeated by audience.)

This moment of silence.

 (Repeated by audience.)

We will be rewarded...

 (Repeated by audience.)

With one humorous detail about his death.

 (Repeated by audience.)

(To an audience member.) It will only be after we have achieved the moment of silence.

 (MIKE *bows his head. We wait for the moment of silence. Yes, we actually wait.)*

After he died, his body disintegrated within six hours.

The point is...

(**MIKE** *walks center stage to where he pantomimed seeing the "no breath holding" sign.*)

After I saw the "no breath holding" sign, I get out of the water. I dry myself with fifteen or twenty of those dish rag-sized YMCA towels. I walk into the locker room, I take off my swim cap, and I pull down my swim trunks and I sit down on the bench.

(**MIKE** *sits on the stool with the posture of the old man from the locker room flashback.*)

I'm reminded of the old man when I was a kid at the YMCA and for the first time in my life I thought, *Maybe he knew something I didn't know.*

He was the oldest man I'd ever seen. He lived a long life. He had taken care of his body. He swam. He had sensitive skin. Here I was, this seven-year-old kid laughing about this old man, but maybe the roadmap to my own maturity was in the veins of this man's testicles.

(*Beat, walking downstage.*)

The old man is dead. And we're all the old man. Or we will be if we're lucky. And any of us could be the man who died holding his breath in the YMCA pool. Or the woman who was killed by a coconut falling on her head. Any of us could be diagnosed with terminal cancer. All we are promised is this moment right now [at the Vivian Beaumont Theater in New York City].

These are the days of us.

And what I want to tell my parents –

(An abrupt cut to black. It's intentionally abrupt, mid-sentence. In darkness the song from the opening plays. Lights come up for bows.)*

End of Play

---

* A license to produce *The Old Man and the Pool* does not include a performance license for any third-party or copyrighted music. Licensees should create an original composition or use music in the public domain. For further information, please see the Music and Third-Party Materials Use Note on page iii.

www.ingramcontent.com/pod-product-compliance
Lightning Source LLC
Chambersburg PA
CBHW070421120726
47909CB00005B/1748